Chair Yoga
for
Seniors

Alex Harper

"For the wise and wonderful elders who continue to inspire us with their perseverance and wisdom, this book is a tribute to your enduring vitality. May it enhance your journey of wellness and joy."

Alex Harper

VIDEO BONUS

Want **FREE BOOKS** for the rest of your LIFE?

Join our VIP club now by scanning the QR code to get **FREE** access to all our future books.

We ONLY send you an email when we launch a NEW BOOK. NO SPAM. Never. Ever!

Just an email with **YOUR 100% OFF COUPON CODE.**

To get your **FREE** lifetime 🎥 **VIDEO ACCESS** 🎥 to our invigorating **CHAIR YOGA EXERCISES** just scan the QR code above or enter this link https://bit.ly/chair-yoga-videocourse into your search browser.

Get ready to elevate your fitness journey!

TABLE OF CONTENTS

Introduction --7

Chapter 1: Unlocking the Power of Chair Yoga --------------------------------9

The Benefits of Chair Yoga-- 9

Principles of Chair Yoga --10

Chapter 2: Breathing --- 14

Unlock the power of breathing to enhance overall health and reduce stress ---14

Chapter 3: Preparation --- 17

Chapter 4: Exercises --- 22

Warm-Up Exercises --22

Beginner Exercises --31

Intermediate Exercises--42

Advanced Exercises --53

Toning Exercises --67

Cardio Exercises--74

Meditation Exercises --80

Chapter 5: 28 Day Challenge --- 92

Structured to gradually increase difficulty, ensuring steady progress-----------80

Bonus Chapter 1: Meditation --109

Learn techniques to calm your mind and improve mental clarity ------------ 109

Bonus Chapter 2: Sleep --112

Discover strategies for achieving deep, restful sleep every night ------------- 112

3 Secret Bonuses --118

Conclusion--117

References--119

BEFORE YOU BEGIN

Hey, thank you for picking up this book! I have poured my heart into writing it to ensure safety and accuracy. All of the written content here has been fact-checked and cited prior to making definitive claims. The information within the pages of this book aims to guide and support women who love Chair Yoga, and those who desire to venture into the practice.

I would highly appreciate it if you left a review after reading this book. As a new author, I enjoy getting to know the transformations you have experienced through my books. Your reviews will help me produce more beneficial content and motivate me to continue the work that I do. Enjoy your read!

INTRODUCTION

Have you ever wondered why you feel fatigued and devoid of energy to keep moving from one place to another? Well, you have found the right book to address all your shortcomings. The latest scientific breakthroughs have made it possible for us to see through the phenomena that were opaque to humanity until the preceding century, opening our eyes to the importance of exercise and yoga.

People with chronic ailments must perform exercises and yoga so their muscles can retain elasticity and they can perform daily tasks with considerable ease. Exercises and yoga postures coupled with meditation and good sleep patterns can make life more fruitful because they all help in maintaining high levels of serotonin (the happy hormone) in the bloodstream.

I am Alex Harper, a certified fitness expert who has helped hundreds of people achieve their fitness goals. As we grow older, the importance of committing to a life that is not thwarted by ailing muscles cannot be overlooked, and therefore, I have combined my decade of experience into a book that can address the needs of seniors.

Fitness knows no age boundary, and we can all stay fit throughout our lives. The key is to find the motivation that can keep us from deviating off course. As a fitness expert, I am familiar with the struggles that seniors face in realizing their fitness goals. I have tons of experience guiding people to sculpt the figure of their dreams, thereby boosting their confidence and morale. Hundreds and thousands of satisfied clients can speak to the work I put into training my clients.

Chair yoga is unique because it can be practiced by fitness enthusiasts of all ages. Moreover, it's not just for those who can't do traditional yoga; you can commit to a program of chair yoga even if you just don't want to do yoga on a mat on the floor. There is a way to achieve your goals comfortably, and you have all the right in the world to chase your goals in the way you deem fit.

So, strap tight for a journey that takes you to the depths of your inner self!

CHAPTER 1: UNLOCKING THE POWER OF CHAIR YOGA

"Yoga is not about touching your toes,
it's about what you learn on the way down."

–Jigar Gor

Chair yoga is a form of yoga that helps you slide into your daily exercise and meditation regimen with considerable ease. Granted, most of us tend to rethink our dedication to getting lean and having a tranquil state of mind when we realize we need to do tons of preparatory work. However, using a chair that can be placed anywhere in your home to do yoga exercises has changed how people approach yoga.

Indubitably, yoga has become more accessible. Chair yoga helps build strength, resilience, and coordination in seniors, who may struggle to achieve the same through traditional yoga. Seniors find it very easy to do yoga on a chair, as it helps with their mobility. They can ease into their chair yoga regimen gradually.

The Benefits of Chair Yoga

The major benefit of chair yoga is that it helps keep the parts of your body that you're not meant to move in position so you can focus on the other parts of your body that you're meant to move. Seniors mostly suffer from chronic medical conditions and mobility issues stemming from arthritis. This calls for an exercise routine that is relatively easy to adopt for seniors. Doing these exercises in a sitting position in a comfy chair makes it easy for the elderly to focus on the correct movement of the limbs. The following are some benefits of chair yoga:

- Augmented strength and flexibility
- Improved balance
- Better cardiovascular health
- Reduced tendency to fall and improved mood

Improved Mobility, Strength, and Flexibility

Practicing a pose daily strengthens your body and makes your muscles flexible. The muscle fibers show better tensile strength, allowing you to perform tasks more efficiently, without feeling pain or fatigue.

Improved Balance and Reduced Tendency to Fall

The ability to balance yourself diminishes with age, but yoga can make you more aware of your limits. It helps you hone your senses and balance your body. As pain and discomfort start to dampen, your balance and agility improve.

Better Cardiovascular Health and Posture

Daily physical activity makes the heart more efficient at pumping blood all around the body and fortifies the muscles, which improves posture. Furthermore, the tendons holding the muscles and bones together become stronger as do the ligaments. As such, the muscles can lift heavier weights and perform more tasks. Seniors can become more agile, especially when they become more invested in their daily activities and hobbies, such as gardening and wildcrafting.

Principles of Chair Yoga

Principles help us understand what we are doing and why we are doing it. Without principles, repeated actions can easily become meaningless, and we will become unmotivated and bored. Chair Yoga has a set of principles that it operates on, and understanding them will help you reap the most benefits out of your practice. The core principles in Yoga are alignment, stability, and breathwork.

Alignment and Stability

According to the Bone Health and Osteoporosis Foundation (n.d.), alignment refers to how the spine, head, shoulders, pelvis, hips, knees, and ankles line up with each other. Improper alignment and form can lead to uncomfortable conditions like slipped discs in the lower back. Below are some simple alignment steps that you can practice while performing Chair Yoga to ensure that you avoid injuries and enhance your workout.

Neutral Spine

Your back has three curves: one in the neck, one in the thoracic region (middle back), and one in the lower back. Maintaining a neutral spine means that all three of those regions are aligned. To find this alignment, lie down on your back, then bend your knees with your feet flat on the mat.

Rest your body on the mat, ensuring that you have no tension or tightness in any area, then tuck your pelvis by drawing your navel toward your spine. There should be little space between the mat and your back; if there isn't, tilt the pelvic region upwards away from the floor.

Shoulder Position

Maintain good shoulder alignment by pulling your scapulae (shoulder blades) downward. Release any tension in your shoulders by inhaling as you lift them, then exhaling as you gently lower them back down.

Head Alignment

Pay extra attention to your head alignment during Chair Yoga because we normally tend to keep it shrugged, bent, or however we feel like. To make sure your head is aligned with your spine, shoulders, and pelvis, imagine an invisible line is tied to the center of your head and is pulling your head upward.

Allow this invisible line to pull your head until your neck is extended and no longer curved. This shouldn't make you feel uncomfortable, but if it does, slowly drop your eyes down to the floor and let your head follow until you no longer feel any discomfort or tension.

Pelvic Alignment

Tuck your tailbone inward and engage your lower abdominal muscles to stabilize your pelvis. To make sure that your pelvis is in alignment with your spine, stand with your back against a wall. Next, put your hand in the space that your back makes with the wall. Then, tuck your pelvis in, lift your chest, and engage your shoulder blades—all while making sure your rib cage is expanded.

Once you've done so, check if the space between your lower back and the wall is minimal to none. That will also depend on the level of your strength and flexibility, so don't fret if you find that there is still a lot of space when you do that. As you continue practicing Chair Yoga, you will get more flexible.

Hip and Knee Alignment

Your hips also have to remain in alignment with your knees. Align them by maintaining a parallel position between your hips and knees. You can also test your alignment by standing hip-width apart and avoiding bending your knees or locking them in too tightly. Don't let your knees collapse inward or push them too far outward.

Strengthening Core Stability

A strong core will help you enhance stability when practicing Chair Yoga. It will also help improve your posture and balance. If you find it difficult to maintain body alignment and stability, focus on building strength in your core muscles.

The stronger your core, the more precise your movements will be; and for us who want a better midsection, a strong core will give you those washboard abs!

CHAPTER 2: BREATHING

"Breath is the bridge which connects life to consciousness, which unites your body to your thoughts."

—Thich Nhat Hanh

The importance of breathing in yoga is something that cannot be overlooked. Breathwork plays a critical role in activating the systems within the body and brings about meaningful change. With the correct type of breathwork, you can bypass the mind and enter a different state of awareness. Breathwork helps you plunge deep into your inner self, where healing takes place and love resides. Your spirit also plays a critical role here. This chapter sheds light on a few breathwork techniques you can incorporate into your meditation routine to gain a deeper sense of your inner self.

Nadi Shodhana Pranayama (Alternate Nostril Breathing)

"Nadi" is a subtle energy channel within the body that can get obstructed for many reasons, but you can unclog this channel using breathwork. The steps to do this are listed below:

1. Sit calmly with your spine in its natural curved position. Place your hands on your knees with the palms facing the ceiling.

2. Place your index and middle fingers between your eyebrows and your ring and little finger on the left nostril. Place your thumb on your right nostril. The ring finger, little finger, and thumb function as plugs that open and close the nostrils.

3. Plug your right nostril and breathe in from your left nostril. Then, plug your left nostril and breathe in from your right nostril.

4. Complete nine such rounds of breathing with your eyes closed.

Bhramari Pranayama (Bee Breath)

The sound of bee humming has great power, as it helps you feel relaxed. This exercise helps imitate bee humming to replicate the same energy within your body.

1. Sit comfortably on your chair and plug your ears with your index fingers.

2. Exhale as much air as you can and make low-pitched humming sounds.

3. Inhale and lift your fingers so your ears are opened. Keep your eyes closed throughout this exercise. You can perform bee breath up to nine times daily.

Dirga Pranayama (Three-Part Breath)

1. Place both hands on your belly such that a few fingers lie below your belly button. Notice the movement.

2. Take deep breaths and try to deepen the airflow so that your lower abdomen feels distended. Continue this phase for a sequence of five breaths.

3. Keep your right hand in its place and move your left hand toward the outer edge of your ribs. Take deep breaths, but this time, expand your belly before your ribs. Continue this motion for five consecutive calming breaths.

4. Now, slide your left hand onto your chest and take deep breaths. This time, expand your chest. These are called grounding breaths.

5. Repeat this cycle for as long as you feel comfortable.

Sama Vritti Pranayama (Equal Breathing)

This exercise can be practiced by lying on your back as well if you do not feel like doing it while sitting on a chair.

1. Find your breath. Gently breathe in and out of your lungs using diaphragmatic breathing so you breathe in and out with no movement in your chest.

2. Set your pace and breathe in and out for a specific count, such as four counts.

3. Repeat this cycle for up to 10 minutes.

Bhastrika Pranayama (Bellows Breath)

Exhale as much air as you can and inhale quickly using diaphragmatic breathing.

The gist of this exercise is to use the muscles of your diaphragm and the abdomen to force out as much air as possible and inhale the highest volume of air as quickly as possible. This exercise is very similar to equal breathing, except that you do not need to follow special sitting instructions to perform the breathing movements. You only need to be able to detect the muscles in your body that need to undergo contraction and use them to do the breathwork that is a part of this kind of yoga.

CHAPTER 3: PREPARATION

The body benefits from movement,
and the mind benefits from stillness.

–Sakyong Mipham

The succinct saying above encapsulates the state of mind that best utilizes the benefits of yoga. You need to be able to reap as much benefit as you can from your yoga practices. There is a benefit galore that comes with the right frame of mind with which you carry yourself into the world of yoga. Therefore, you need to maximize the advantage that can be reaped from your dedication to yoga. As you strap yourself tight for an adventure into your realm of yoga, do not forget to prepare the room and its surroundings, as this prepares your mind for your yoga practices.

Choosing the Right Chair, Equipment, and Clothing

The Choice of Chair

First, you need to find a sturdy chair on which to perform your yoga exercises. A sturdy chair with good and strong pedestals is an absolute necessity, and this is especially true for seniors. Yoga involves different kinds of movements wherein your body weight may shift from one edge of the chair to another. Therefore, you need to have a chair that can withstand the weight of your body as it supports it.

A wide range of chairs are available for you to choose from. Try to go to a shop that boasts having all kinds of chairs suitable for all purposes. For yoga, you need preferably a wooden chair with a slightly reclined backrest for the free movement of limbs. This way, you can lean back whenever you need a break between exercises.

Place a yoga mat beneath the chair before you start chair yoga. The mat helps the chair remain stable on the floor.

Moreover, try to push down on the chair when you buy it from the store so that you know it is stable and does not tilt along with your weight toward one side.

Clothing

Clothing is crucial when wanting to feel comfortable in general, and especially when practicing yoga. Getting into the right gear for your yoga session has immense benefits. Wear comfortable clothing that does not interfere with your movement as you transition between poses. Tight jeans and shorts tend to restrict you as you move your limbs. Try to go for loose clothing, but do not wear too baggy clothes, as they have the same restrictive effect on your movement.

Clear your surroundings of any obstacles that could interfere with the movement of your limbs. Place your chair in an open area.

Warm-Up and Cool-Down Exercises

Warming up your body enhances the benefits of yoga. Warm-up exercises primarily comprise exercises that help prepare your muscles for the strain they'll be experiencing. This helps your muscles perform yoga easily, reducing the chances of injury. While yoga comprises low-intensity movements, stretching your muscle fibers beforehand helps them move better and more comfortably.

Cooling down exercises bear similar importance and must be done after you finish your yoga session. These exercises allow you to transition into a state of rest that comprises muscle recovery. Your muscles are filled with lactic acid, especially after strenuous workouts. While yoga does not incur an oxygen debt, you must still commit to a cooling-down phase because it helps your muscles recover swiftly. These exercises consist of different techniques of meditation exercises, promoting relaxation and mental clarity alongside physical recovery.

How to Progress Week by Week

Making progress should be one of your goals in your practice. However, it is easy for us to feel stressed and pressured over workout goals because of the unrealistic beauty standards that the media feeds us. Maintaining your Chair Yoga practice as a way to get fit and get in touch with your body requires a strategy involving progressive exercises that don't put unrealistic pressure on yourself. Below are a few ways to make gentle progress in your Yoga practice.

Listening To Your Body's Signals

Pay Attention to Discomfort and Pain

Contrary to popular belief, pain and discomfort are not signs of a great workout session. Muscle soreness and pain are usually signs that you did not stretch or that you challenged yourself beyond what you were able to handle. Although it's wise to challenge yourself so that you can grow, overdoing it will actually deter your progress because you will have to pause your practice for a longer period of time to allow your muscles to heal.

Pain during your practice is also a sign that you are overworking your muscles in an unhealthy way. Pay attention to pain and discomfort, then stop to rest and check your posture and alignment to avoid injuries.

Monitor Your Breathing

Breathing is the force of life within our bodies that activates muscles and helps us shift into powerful states. Engaging in challenging movements can distract you from breathing steadily, and you may start to feel lightheaded. Always refocus on your breathing to make sure that you have enough oxygen flowing to your muscles and that you are mindful of the present moment.

Be Mindful of Fatigue and Energy Levels

During exercises, you may experience two thresholds. The first one is the mental threshold. At that stage, you will be faced with your own mental blocks and an inner critic telling you to just stop. The second threshold is your body's actual tolerance level. At that stage, you will feel fatigued, and if you push past your tolerance levels forcefully, you will get lightheaded and may injure yourself.

Pay attention to your body and your mind in order to know which threshold you are at, so you can gently support yourself either by encouraging yourself to push past mental blocks or by stopping and adding another set of movements during another Chair Yoga session.

Aspects of Yoga to Avoid

We are all likely to overstretch, so you need to check your body's limits and only twist or stretch as far as your body can bear. Weakened muscles can be subject to tears, and the pain that follows can be unbearable.

Holding a pose for too long might seem very tempting, but again, do not burden your body with something it cannot bear. Hold a pose only for as long as your body can bear the force exerted by the pose.

Seniors must avoid deep backbends, as these movements involve the back and can exert a force that is too intense to be borne in old age. Also, inversions must be avoided. These are movements wherein the head sinks below the heart's position, which can result in an undue detrimental impact on cardiovascular health.

Safe Practice

Listen to your body and learn your own limits. Do not subject your body to overexertion. Do not try to push your limits too early. Work within your limits and slowly push yourself to perform more poses or hold some poses for longer periods.

Your yoga practice must be consistent. Do not fall prey to the idea of doing more one day, as this can be very exhausting for you and result in you skipping yoga altogether the next day. Finally, remember to hydrate!

CHAPTER 4: EXERCISES

WARM-UP EXERCISES

1. CHAIR CAT-COW STRETCH

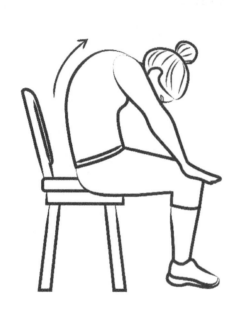 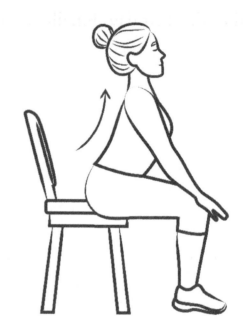

Purpose:

This dynamic stretch promotes flexibility and mobility in the spine. It helps to relieve tension in the back and neck. The flowing movement between Cat and Cow Pose also stimulates the organs in the belly, improving digestion.

Execution:

- Sit on the edge of the chair with your feet flat on the floor.
- Place your hands on your knees or thighs.

- As you inhale, arch your back, open your chest, and lift your gaze towards the ceiling for Cow Pose.
- As you exhale, round your back, draw your belly button towards your spine, and let your head drop forward for Cat Pose.
- Continue to flow between these two poses for several breaths, moving with the rhythm of your breath.

2. NECK ROLL

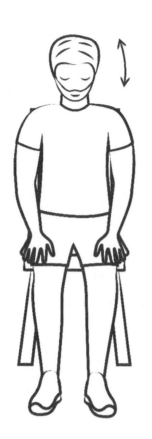
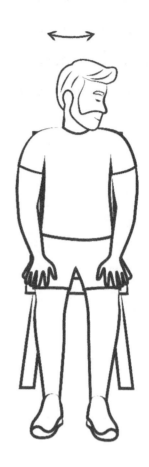

Purpose:

Seated neck rolls not only enhance neck flexibility, but it also paves the way for improved posture, fostering overall spinal health.

Execution:

- Sit on the edge of the chair with your feet flat on the floor.
- Place your hands on your knees or thighs.
- Inhale deeply and gently lower your chin towards your chest, feeling a subtle stretch in the back of your neck.
- Slowly rotate your head to the right, aiming to bring your right ear closer to your right shoulder without straining.

- Exhale and guide your chin back to your chest in a controlled motion.
- Inhale and gently turn your head to the left, attempting to bring your left ear towards your left shoulder with ease.
- Exhale and return your chin to your chest, finalizing one full neck rotation.

3. SHOULDER SHRUGS

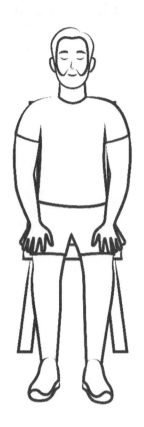 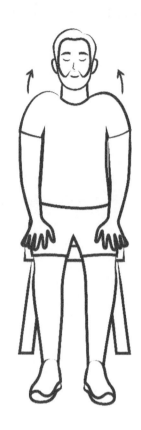

Purpose:

This warm-up exercise reduces tension in your traps, neck, and shoulders, preparing you fully for upcoming exercises.

Execution:

- Sit upright with your feet shoulder-distance apart.
- Inhale and lift your shoulders towards your ears, holding them there briefly.
- Exhale and release the tension by slowly lowering your shoulders away from your ears.
- Repeat the movement 5 to 10 times.

4. ARM CIRCLES

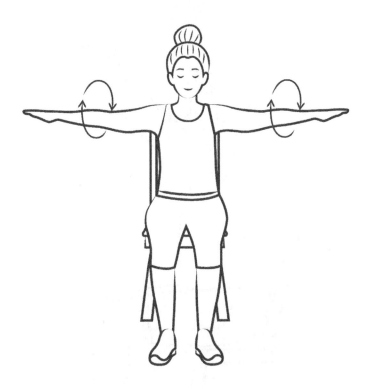

Purpose:

Arm Circles improves flexibility and range of motion in the upper body. These circular motions also increase heart rate which improves cardiovascularity.

Execution:

- Sit on a chair with your feet shoulders distance apart.
- Slowly raise both arms out to the sides at shoulder height.
- Begin making small circular motions with both arms simultaneously.
- Bring your hands onto your knees after completing 10 - 15 repetitions.
- Relax for a few breaths and then repeat the exercise, but reverse the direction of the circles this time; if you initially made clockwise circles, try counterclockwise this time.
- Make sure to control your breathing and avoid any jerky movements.

5. SEATED URDHVA HASTASANA

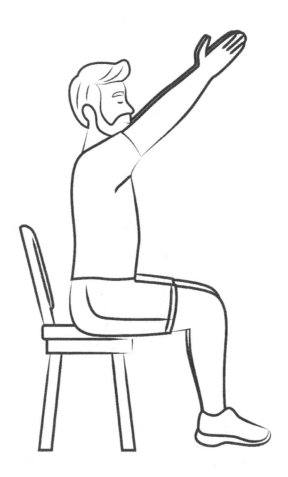

Purpose:

The focus of this pose is to build range in your shoulder joints while using your arms as a downward driver to load and unload your upper back.

Execution:

- Sit upright on the chair. Ideally, slightly away from the backrest so that you have to use your postural muscles and core strength.
- On the inhale, raise your arms towards the ceiling while drawing your shoulder blades together and downwards.
- Imagine that you have an invisible pencil that you're trying to gently grip between your shoulder blades as you move.

- If you feel stiff and can't raise the arms all the way up, then just go as high as you can.

- Hold the arms there for a count of 20 seconds and take several controlled breaths in and out while maintaining your posture and drawing in your abs.

- Slowly lower your arms until they are at your sides. Repeat for 5 repetitions.

6. LEG PENDULUMS

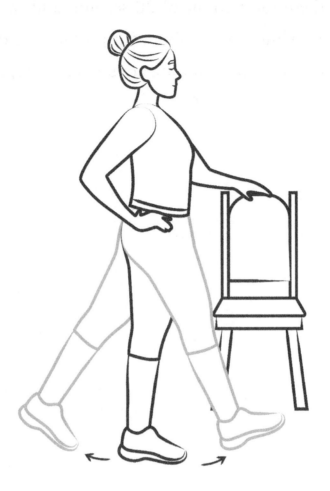

Purpose:

This dynamic stretching exercise helps loosen up your muscles, preparing you for your chair yoga session.

Execution:

- Place one hand on a wall or hold the back of a chair for balance. Stand on one leg (keeping it straight). Swing the other leg (also straight) forward and backward 10 times.
- Switch your legs and repeat the same for the other leg.

BEGINNER EXERCISES

7. STANDING WIND RELEASE

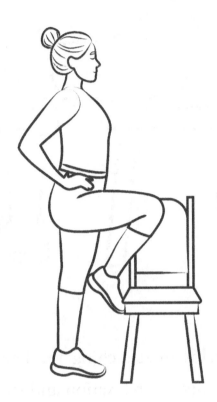

Purpose:

This exercise helps in improving balance, strengthens the standing leg, and promotes hip mobility.

Execution:

- Stand beside your chair, holding onto the backrest for support.
- Shift your weight onto one leg and as you exhale, bring the opposite knee towards your chest, holding it with your hand.
- Inhale to release the leg back to the floor.
- Exhale to bring the knee towards the chest again.
- Repeat on the other side.

8. CHAIR CHILD'S POSE

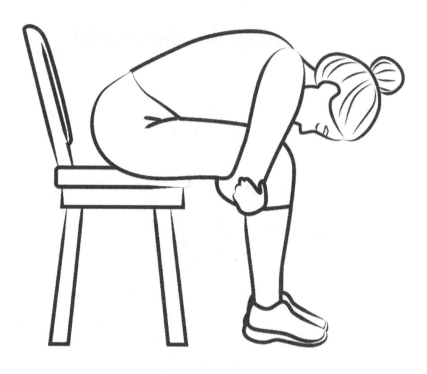

Purpose:

Chair Child's Pose helps in stretching the back, hips, and thighs. It is a restorative pose that promotes relaxation and stress relief. The pose also aids in improving flexibility in the hips and spine.

Execution:

- Sit on the edge of the chair with your feet flat on the floor.
- As you exhale, hinge at your hips and fold forward, extending your arms in front of you and resting your torso on your thighs.
- Hug your thighs with your arms and hold this position.
- Slowly come back up to a seated position as you inhale.

9. SEATED TWIST

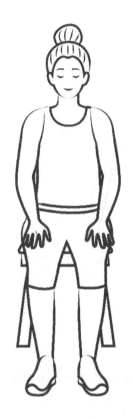 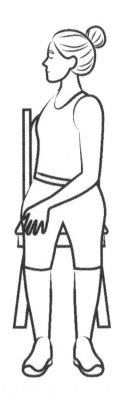

Purpose:

The Seated Twist helps in increasing spinal flexibility and relieving tension along the spine.. This pose can also help in stimulating circulation and improving overall posture.

Execution:

- Sit on the chair with your feet flat on the floor, hip-width apart. Sit tall, elongating your spine.
- As you inhale, lengthen your spine further.
- As you exhale, twist your torso to the right, placing your left hand on the outside of your right knee and your right hand on the back of the chair.
- With each inhale, lengthen your spine, and with each exhale, deepen your twist.
- Hold for a few breaths, then slowly come back to center and repeat on the other side.

10. SEATED FORWARD BEND

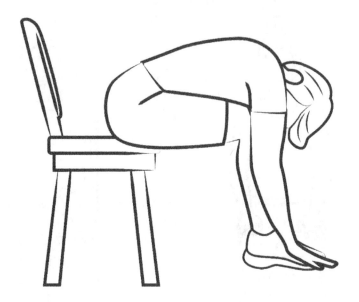

Purpose:

The Seated Forward Bend stretches the spine and helps in relieving tension in the back. It also stretches the hamstrings and can aid in improving digestion by massaging the abdominal organs.

Execution:

- Sit on the edge of the chair with your feet flat on the floor, hip-width apart.
- Keep your spine long and your shoulders relaxed away from your ears.
- Inhale deeply, and as you exhale, hinge at your hips and fold forward, bringing your chest towards your thighs.
- You can rest your hands on your legs, the floor, or on a block, depending on your flexibility.
- Let your head hang heavy, or rest it on a support if needed.
- Hold this position for a few breaths, then slowly come back up to a seated position as you inhale.

11. SEATED SIDE STRETCH

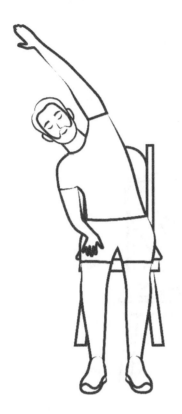 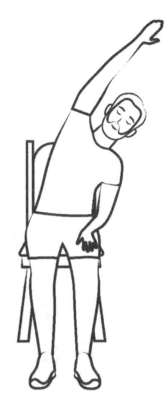

Purpose:

This stretch opens up the side body, improving flexibility and breathing capacity. It also helps in relieving tension along the spine and in the shoulders.

Execution:

- Sit comfortably on the chair with your feet flat on the floor. Keep your spine straight and shoulders relaxed.
- Inhale deeply, and as you exhale, gently lean to the right side, sliding your right hand down the side of the chair.
- Extend your left arm overhead, reaching towards the right side, keeping your arm in line with your ear.
- Keep your chest open and your gaze towards the ceiling or straight ahead.
- Hold for a few breaths, then slowly come back to center as you inhale.
- Repeat on the other side.

12. CHAIR LUNGE POSE

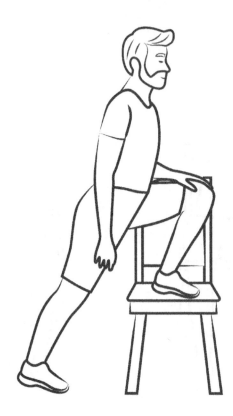

Purpose:

Chair Lunge Pose strengthens the legs and stretches the hips and thighs. It also enhances balance and stability.

Execution:

- Start by standing a little distance away from the chair. Place your left foot on the seat of the chair.
- Bend your left knee and lower your body towards the floor, keeping a right angle in your left knee.
- Extend your arms overhead or keep them rested against your waist, keeping your shoulders relaxed.
- Hold the pose for a few breaths, feeling the stretch.
- Slowly return to the starting position and switch sides.

13.   SEATED CACTUS POSE

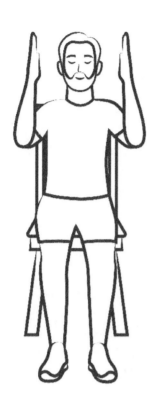 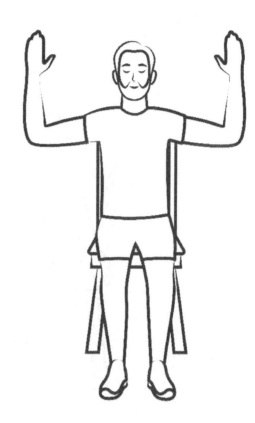

Purpose:

This exercise helps to open up the chest and shoulders, which can become tight from hunching over. It also helps to strengthen the muscles between the shoulder blades, improving posture and stability.

Execution:

- Sit tall in your chair, feet flat on the floor. Extend your arms out to the sides at shoulder height.
- Bend your elbows to a 90-degree angle, with your palms facing forward.
- As you inhale, squeeze your shoulder blades together, opening up your chest.
- As you exhale, bring your elbows towards each other in front of you without collapsing your chest.
- Continue this opening and closing movement for several breaths.

14. COBRA POSE

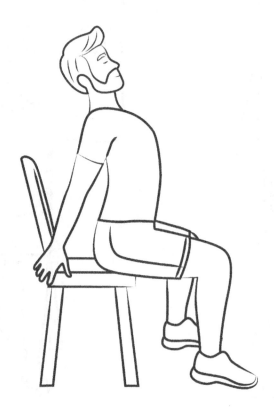

Purpose:

The Chair Cobra Pose is a gentle seated backbend designed to open the chest and stretch the upper back.

Execution:

- Sit at the front edge of your chair, ensuring your feet are flat on the ground and hip-distance apart. Lengthen your spine, ensuring your back is straight.
- Place your hands on the back of the chair, holding it firmly.
- As you inhale, lift your chest towards the ceiling, arching your back slightly. Allow your gaze to move upwards, feeling an opening in the chest.
- Maintain this arched position, feeling the stretch in your upper back and chest. Ensure your neck remains relaxed and avoid straining it.
- Exhale and return to the starting position.

15. HUMBLE WARRIOR POSE

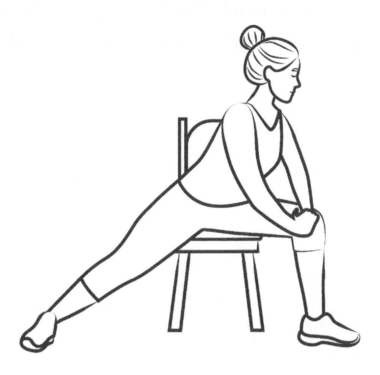

Purpose:

This variation of the traditional Humble Warrior Pose targets the legs, hips, arms, chest, rib cage, shoulders, spine, and core muscles, offering a comprehensive stretch and engagement for these areas.

Execution:

- Begin by ensuring you're seated comfortably on a chair with your spine straight.
- Turn your front foot (the one closest to the chair) to point directly forward, and angle your back foot slightly inwards, approximately 45 degrees.
- Bend your front knee, making sure it aligns directly over your ankle. Ensure your knee points in the same direction as your front foot.
- Adjust your seated position slightly to accommodate more of your forward leg on the chair. Place your hands on your front knee with fingers interlocked.
- Keep the elbows bent and pointed to the sides.

- Keep the chest broad and lifted, with a gentle twist and a slight forward bend.

- Ensure the chin is aligned with the chest and slightly tucked in. Keep the shoulders broad. Look downwards. Exhale as you bend forward.

- Hold the position for a few breaths and release. Repeat on the opposite side.

16. MOUNTAIN POSE

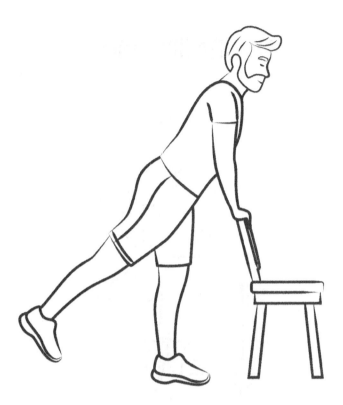

Purpose:

This exercise challenges stability and engages the core while also strengthening your hamstrings, glutes and enhancing hip mobility.

Execution:

- Stand in front of a chair, ensuring your feet are hip-width apart and your spine is straight.
- Slightly bend your torso forward and find your balance by holding onto the chair.
- Raise one leg backward, keeping it straight.
- Hold this position briefly, feeling the engagement in the leg and the stretch in the hip flexors. Lower your leg back to the ground, returning to the starting position. Repeat the same steps with the other leg.

INTERMEDIATE EXERCISES

17. STANDING TREE

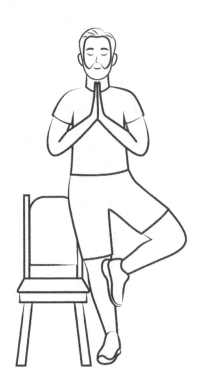

Purpose:

Standing Tree Pose enhances balance and stability. It strengthens the legs, ankles, and feet, and promotes good posture.

Execution:

- Stand beside your chair for support, with your feet hip-width apart.
- Start with your palms facing each other or keep your hands in prayer position at your chest. Use the chair as a support for your right leg.
- Now place your left foot on your right thigh creating a reverse "4".
- Keep your core engaged, shoulders relaxed, and gaze fixed on a point in above of you.
- Hold the pose for a few breaths, then slowly release and switch sides.

18. STANDING HASTASAN

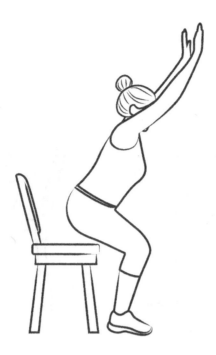

Purpose:

Chair Pose strengthens the legs, glutes, and lower back. It also engages the core and promotes better posture.

Execution:

- Stand with your feet hip-width apart, toes pointing forward.
- Extend your arms overhead with your palms facing each other.
- As you exhale, bend your knees and lower your hips back and down as if you were going to sit in a chair. You can keep your arms raised or rest them on the back of the chair.
- Keep your chest lifted and shoulders relaxed, and avoid arching your lower back.
- Hold the pose for a few breaths, engaging your thighs and glutes.
- Inhale as you slowly stand back up to the starting position.

19. PRAYING SPINAL TWIST

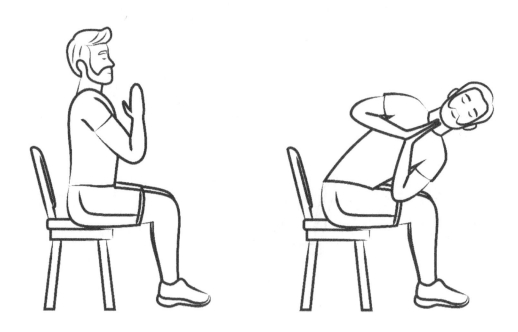

Purpose:

This pose helps to stretch and open the shoulders and chest. It also massages and stimulates the abdominal organs which can aid in digestion and help to relieve minor back pain.

Execution:

- Sit comfortably on your chair with your feet flat on the floor, hip-width apart.
- Sit tall, extending your spine towards the ceiling.
- As you inhale, lengthen your spine and as you exhale, begin to twist to your left from the base of your spine.
- Bring the palms of your hands together to chest level. Use each inhalation to lengthen your spine, and each exhalation to deepen the twist.
- Keep your chin in line with your chest to ensure a gentle neck.
- Hold for a few breaths, then slowly unwind on an exhalation and repeat on the other side.

20. CHAIR PIGEON POSE

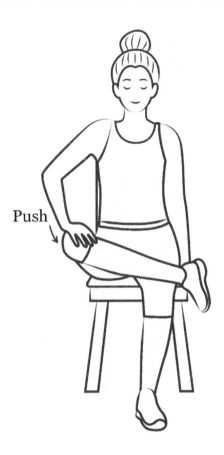

Push

Purpose:

Chair Pigeon Pose opens up the hips and stretches the thighs and glutes. It also helps in relieving tension and tightness in the lower body.

Execution:

- Sit on the edge of the chair with your feet flat on the floor.
- Keep your spine tall and your shoulders relaxed.
- Lift your right leg and place your right ankle on your left thigh, just above the knee, forming a figure 4 with your legs.
- Flex your right foot to protect your knee. (If this position feels comfortable, you can hinge at the hips and fold forward slightly to deepen the stretch.)
- Hold this position for a few breaths, then slowly release and switch legs.

21.   DANCER POSE

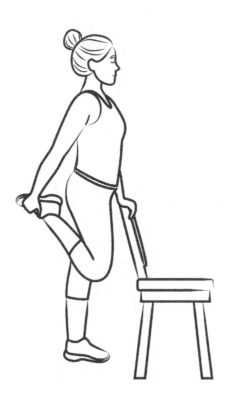

Purpose:

Dancer Pose challenges balance, strengthens the standing leg, and stretches the shoulders, chest, and thighs.

Execution:

-   Stand next to your chair, holding onto the backrest for support with your left hand.
-   Shift your weight onto your left foot.
-   Bend your right knee, bringing your right heel towards your buttocks.
-   Reach back with your right hand to grasp the inside of your right foot or ankle.
-   As you inhale, lift your right foot up towards the ceiling, extending it behind you as you lean slightly forward.
-   Keep your chest lifted and gaze forward.
-   Hold for a few breaths, then slowly release and switch sides.

22. CHAIR EAGLE POSE

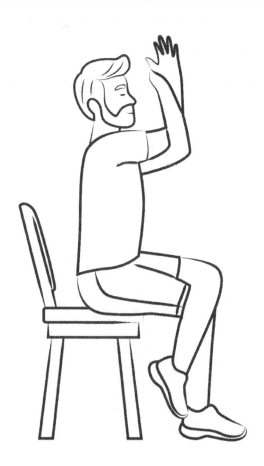

Purpose:

The chair eagle improves muscle tone, circulation, and flexibility.

Execution:

- Sit upright on your chair with your feet hip distance apart.
- Cross your left leg over your right and hook your left foot back around your right ankle in a winding motion. If you don't quite have the range for this yet, take your left leg to a point where you feel comfortable.
- Raise your arms in front of you and cross your right arm over your left. Fold at the elbows so that both your arms point upward. (The goal is to wind your arms around themselves until your palms touch together).

- Just like with your legs, if you don't quite have the range for this yet, take it to the point that you feel a comfortable stretch.
- Now activate your core muscles, lift your chest, and breathe normally.
- Hold the pose for 30 to 60 seconds.
- Return to your start position before repeating the pose on the opposite side.

23. HUMBLE KING ARTHUR'S POSE

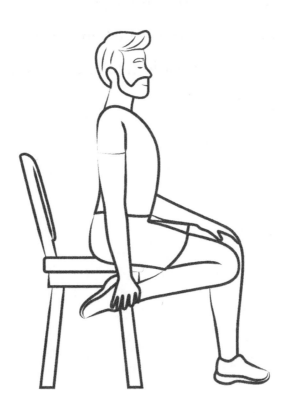

Purpose:

King Arthur's pose focuses on core stability, as well as knee and ankle range of movement.

Execution:

- Sit upright on the right side of your chair, slightly away from the back rest, with your feet hip distance apart.
- Brace your body, focusing on keeping your hips level and your feet planted on the ground.
- Bend your right knee until your foot has lifted off the floor. Reach down with your right arm and gently pull your foot towards your hips while pointing your toes.

- Lift your chest and draw your shoulder blades back and down to complete the pose.. Breathe normally, draw in your abs, and hold form for up to 30 seconds or as long as you comfortably can.

- Just place your foot down to balance when you take a rest. Once you have completed your set, relax the position, take 20 seconds rest, and then practice the pose on your opposite side.

24.   CHAIR WARRIOR POSE

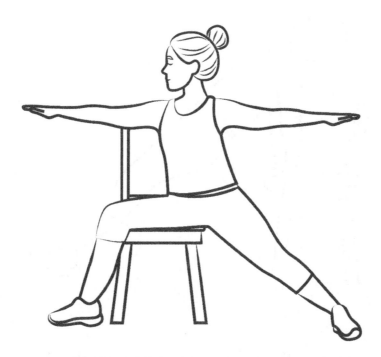

Purpose:

Practice one of the most common yoga exercise in its modified chair version.

Execution:

- Start sitting upright on your chair, slightly over to the left-hand side of the seat.
- Turn to your right and get into a high lunge position, making sure that your right leg is supported by the chair and your left is outstretched behind.
- Turn the foot on your outstretched leg to face forward, making sure that you keep it flat on the ground. Only turn it as far as you can while remaining stable and comfortable. Take a breath in.
- Raise both arms, one in front and one behind, to shoulder height. Open your chest, lengthen your neck, and breathe out as you move.
- Focus on drawing your shoulder blades back and down.
- Hold the pose for 30 seconds while breathing normally.
- Release the pose and switch to opposite side.

25. UPWARD PLANK

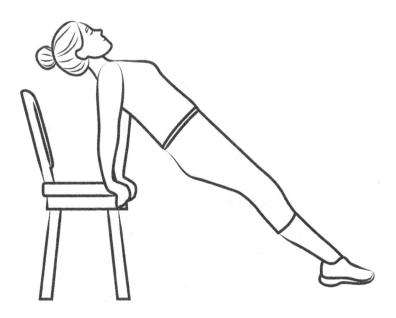

Purpose:

This is a great pose to fix bad posture by strengthening the back and core muscles while enabling you to open your chest.

Execution:

- Sit on a chair with your feet shoulders distance apart. Place your hands directly under your shoulders on the chair with your fingers facing the front of the chair.
- Inhale and slowly extend your legs out to the front until your knees are fully locked out and your toes are pointing towards the ceiling.
- Then, push into the chair with your hands and engage your core to slightly lift yourself off of the chair until your arms are fully locked out. You should aim to get a straight, diagonal line running from your ankles to your head.
- Slightly lift your chest, point your gaze towards the ceiling, and pull your shoulder blades together.
- Hold the pose for a few deep breaths and release by bringing your hips back to the chair and then bringing your legs back to the starting position.

ADVANCED EXERCISES

26. LOW LUNGE POSE

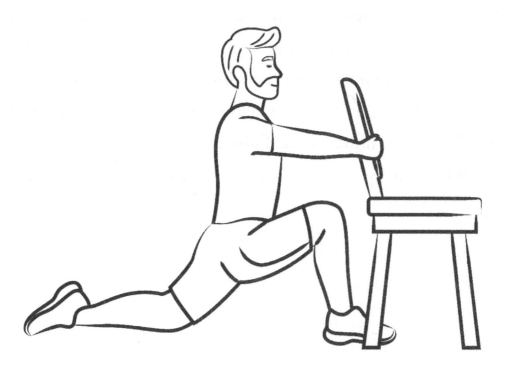

Purpose:

Improves hamstrings, hips, and lower back flexibility, greatly improving your mobility.

Execution:

- Stand a step away from a chair, facing its back, with your feet flat on the ground, shoulder distance apart, and grab the sides of the backrest of the chair firmly.
- As you inhale, slowly move your left foot back to create some distance between your left foot and the chair.
- Your toes should be pointing forward with your heel lifted off of the floor.
- Lower yourself by bending your right leg into a lunge position with your right knee directly above your right ankle.

- Next, extend your left leg straight out behind you until your left knee and the front face of the left foot come into contact with the floor with your toes pointing towards the back.

- Keep your upper body upright with your arms extended in front of you at shoulder height.

- Hold this pose for a few deep breaths before pulling your left leg next to your right leg and then repeating the same steps on the other side by extending your right leg behind you while keeping your left leg bent.

- Hold again for a few deep breaths before pulling your right leg next to your left leg and then slowly lifting yourself into a standing position by pushing into the ground with your legs and pressing down into the chair with your hands.

27. SEATED COW FACE

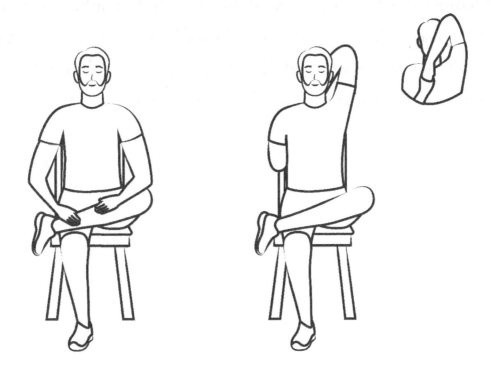

Purpose:

Stretches over ten major muscle groups and enhances shoulder mobility and flexibility.

Execution:

- Sit on a chair with your feet shoulders distance apart.
- Cross your left ankle over your right knee and press down on your left knee to create a deeper stretch.
- Reach your right arm overhead and then bend it at the elbow to place your left hand on your upper back with your left elbow pointing towards the ceiling.
- Next, extend your right arm out to the side and bend it at the elbow to bring your right hand behind your back. Finally, try to grab both hands behind your back. If you are unable to do so, try grabbing a towel or a piece of cloth

in your hands and gently pulling onto it. With practice, you will be able to touch your hands and eventually grab them!

- Remember to sit tall with a straight spine and breathe deeply for 5 breaths before releasing by first letting go of your hands, bringing them back in your lap, and then lifting your right leg, bringing your right foot back to the floor.
- To balance the pose, repeat on the opposite side.

28. BRIDGE POSE

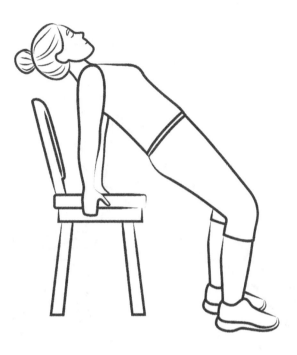

Purpose:

Strengthens the glutes, hamstrings, and lower back muscles, which are crucial for better posture.

Execution:

- Sit on a chair with your feet shoulder-distance apart.
- Place your hands next to you on the sides of the chair for support. Next, press your feet into the ground, engage your core, and push your hands into the seat of the chair to lift your hips off the seat.
- Arch your back slightly by lifting your chest towards the ceiling and bring your shoulder blades closer to each other for stability.
- Your hands should remain directly under your shoulders, holding the weight of your upper body, and your neck should remain in line with your spine to prevent any strain on the neck.
- Hold the pose for 5 breaths before slowly lowering yourself back down to the starting position.

29. CHAIR PLANK

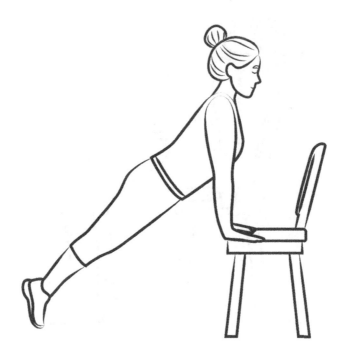

Purpose:

Strengthens arms, shoulders, core, hips, and legs, improving endurance and stamina.

Execution:

- Stand a few steps away from a chair with your feet shoulder distance apart and place the palms of your hands on the top of the backrest of the chair.
- Pull your navel in closer to your spine to engage your core. As you breathe, step back and keep lowering yourself until your head, hips, and toes are in a straight diagonal line with your shoulders directly above your hands.
- Keep your legs engaged to prevent your hips from falling or going too high and keep your spine straight with your neck in line with it to prevent straining it.
- Hold this pose for a few breaths before releasing by walking towards the chair and lifting your torso from your back and pushing the chair with your hands until you stand tall.

- Once you get comfortable with this pose, move to start with your hands on the seat of the chair and repeat the same steps. If moving to the seat of the chair becomes too difficult, try placing your knees on the floor slowly and lift your body to build upper body strength and complete the plank pose.

30. DOWNWARD DOG POSE

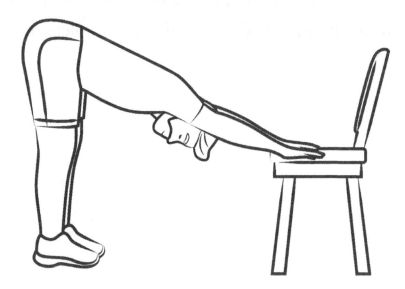

Purpose:

Improves flexibility in the lower back and hamstrings, which helps avoid future injuries.

Execution:

- Stand a few steps away from a chair with your feet on the ground, shoulder distance apart.
- Gently bend forward at your hips to lower your torso closer to the chair and place the palms of your hands on the seat of the chair.
- Next, step back and keep lowering your upper body until your hips, head, and hands are in a straight line, and your upper and lower body form a "V" shape.
- Maintain a slight bend in your knees and press your heels into the floor to lift your hips slightly as you feel a stretch in your hamstrings.
- Hold for a few breaths before releasing by walking towards the chair and lifting your torso by pulling from your back and pressing down with your hands.

31. PIGEON POSE

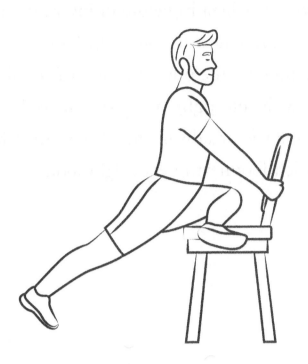

Purpose:

Reduces lower back pain and improves back, hips, and knee mobility.

Execution:

- Stand in front of a chair and lower your upper body slightly to grab the backrest of the chair firmly. Pull your navel in closer to your spine to engage your core.
- Slowly step back and keep lowering yourself until your head, hips, and toes are in a straight diagonal line with your arms in front of you holding the chair.
- Next, bend your left leg to place your right shin on the chair with your left knee pointing out to the side.
- Finally, lift your head by pulling your back and pushing your chest out while letting your hips fall slightly to straighten out your back, parallel to the

backrest of the chair. Keep your neck in line with your spine to prevent straining it, with your gaze directly in front of you.

- Hold this pose for a few breaths before lifting your left shin off of the chair and placing your left foot next to your right foot.

- Then, repeat the pose on the other side by placing the outside of the right shin on the chair with your right knee pointing to the side.

- Hold this pose for a few breaths before lifting your left shin off of the chair and placing your left foot next to your right foot.

32. SEATED SIDE LUNGE

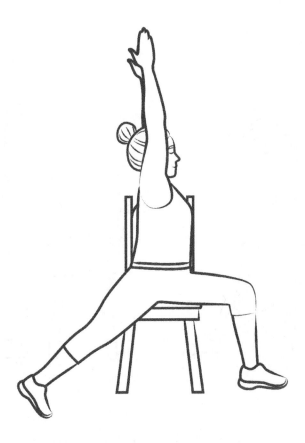

Purpose:

Toning and strengthening your thighs, knees, ankles, and core.

Execution:

- Sit sideways on your chair so that its backrest is next to your left arm.
- Sit toward the edge of the chair so that your left thigh is supported and your right has space to move.
- Hold onto the top of the chair's backrest with your left hand to help support you through the position. Keeping your left foot planted on the floor in front of you with its knee at 90 degrees, lengthen your right leg out behind you, perching on the ball of your right foot.
- Hold for 5 to 10 breaths before repeating on the other side.

33. TRIANGLE POSE

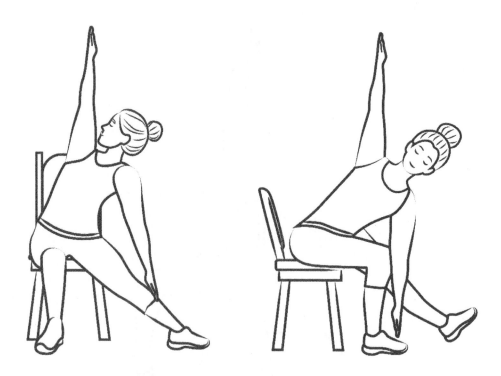

Purpose:

This typical yoga exercise provides deep stretch from your lower back up to your lats and traps.

Execution:

- Sit upright to the left side of the chair, ideally with your left thigh slightly off the chair's seat. Keeping your right leg routed to the floor, extend your left leg out straight at the knee and out at a left angle at the hip.
- Once you are in position, brace your thigh.
- Inhale and raise both arms to shoulder height laterally (to the sides) with your chest open, holding them parallel to the floor.
- Keep your shoulder blades drawn back, and your palms face down.
- Exhale and lean your torso to the left, aiming your left hand toward your outstretched left leg's knee or shin.

- As you reach downward with your left arm, reach upward with your right, rotating your right palm up and aiming toward the ceiling.
- Once in position, turn your head until you can see your right fingertips.
- Hold this position for 8 to 10 breaths.

34.   PUPPY DOG POSE

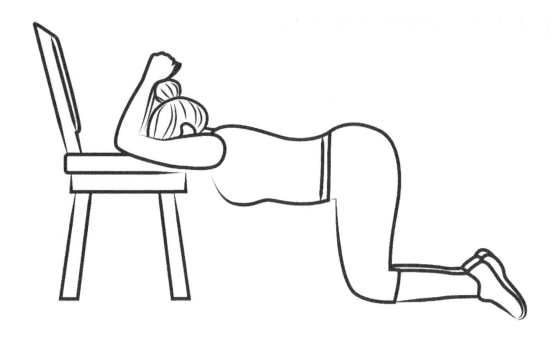

Purpose:

Puppy Dog Pose stretches the spine, lats, and chest, promoting relaxation and a release of tension in the upper body.

Execution:

- Begin by kneeling a few feet away from your chair.
- Hinge at your hips and place your elbows on the chair, keeping your gaze towards the floor.
- Press your chest towards the floor, feeling a stretch in your upper back, lats (sides of the back) and chest while keeping your hips over your knees.
- Hold for several breaths, then slowly return to the starting position

TONING EXERCISES

35.   MODIFIED PUSH UP

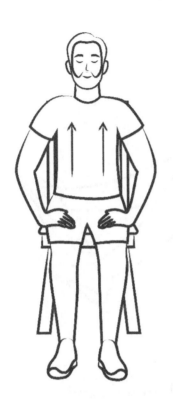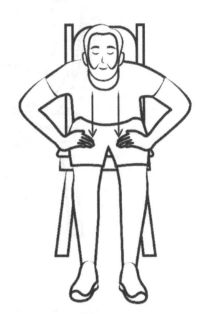

Purpose:

Offers a unique way to work on the upper body muscles.

Executions:

- Sit comfortably on a chair, positioning your legs slightly wider than hip-width apart. Ensure your feet are flat on the ground.
- Rest your hands atop your knees, palms facing down. With a straight back, lean your chest forward towards your legs, going as low as you comfortably can.
- Engage your arms and shoulders to push yourself back to the upright starting position.
- Continue the movement for the desired number of repetitions.

36. LEG SHUFFLE

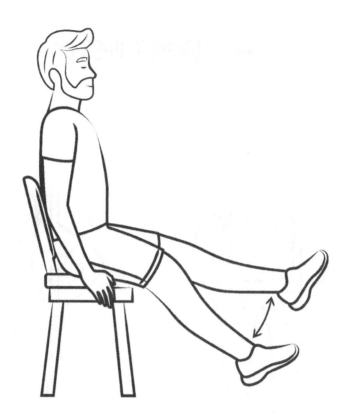

Purpose:

Designed to strengthen the abdominal muscles and core.

Executions:

- Sit at the edge of a sturdy chair, ensuring your back is erect.
- Place your hands on either side of the chair for added stability. Gently lean your upper body backward.
- Lift both feet a few inches off the ground. Begin to shuffle your legs by moving them up and down alternately, as if marching in place.
- Maintain a steady pace and keep the movements controlled, focusing on engaging your lower abs.
- Perform the shuffle for 10-20 repetitions, rest, and repeat for 1-3 sets.

37. LEG RAISES

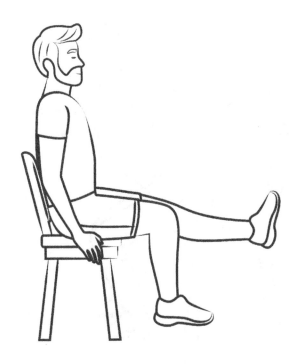

Purpose:

Strengthening and toning the thighs and hip muscles.

Executions:

- Begin by sitting upright on a chair, ensuring your spine is straight and your feet are flat on the ground, hip-width apart.

- Draw your abdomen in, engaging your core muscles to provide stability. Slowly lift one leg, keeping it straight, until it's parallel to the ground or as high as comfortably possible.

- Maintain this position for a couple of breaths, feeling the engagement in your thigh and hip muscles.

- Gently lower your leg back to the starting position. Perform the same steps with the other leg.

- Aim for multiple repetitions on each side.

38. CHAIR SQUAT

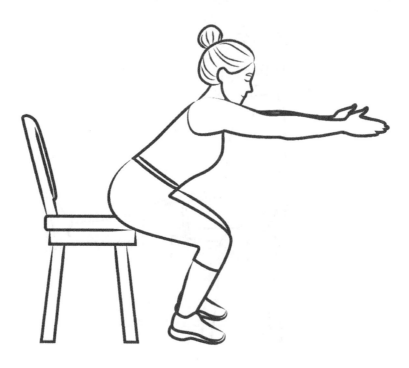

Purpose:

Chair Squats help in strengthening the quadriceps, hamstrings, glutes, and calf muscles.

Execution:

- Begin by sitting on the edge of the chair with your feet flat on the floor, hip-width apart.
- Keep your spine tall and your shoulders relaxed.
- Inhale as you engage your core muscles and push through your heels to stand up, extending your hips and knees.
- Exhale as you slowly lower your body back down, controlling the descent and touching the chair, without sitting down. Make sure your knees are aligned with your toes, and they don't go past your toes as you lower down.
- Repeat the movement for the desired number of repetitions.

39. CHAIR DIPS

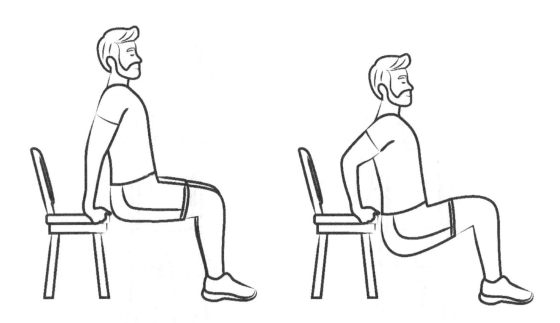

Purpose:

Chair Dips target the triceps, shoulders, and chest muscles. They also challenge your core stability.

Execution:

- Sit on the edge of the chair and grip the front edges of the seat with your hands, knuckles facing forward.
- Walk your feet forward and slide your hips off the chair.
- Lower your body down by bending your elbows, keeping them close to your body.
- Stop when your elbows are at about a 90-degree angle or when you feel a stretch across your chest.
- Push through your hands to straighten your arms and lift your body back to the starting position.
- Repeat for the desired number of repetitions.

40. SHOULDER PRESS

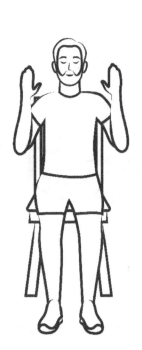
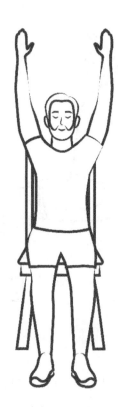

Purpose:

This exercise also promotes better posture by engaging the muscles of the upper back and shoulders.

Execution:

- Sit on the chair with your feet flat on the floor, hip-width apart.
- Hold a pair of lightweight dumbbells or water bottles at shoulder height with your elbows bent, palms facing forward.
- Inhale to prepare, and as you exhale, press the weights overhead, extending your arms fully.
- Inhale as you slowly lower the weights back down to shoulder height.
- Repeat the movement for the desired number of repetitions.

41.   CHAIR SUPPORTED CALF RAISES

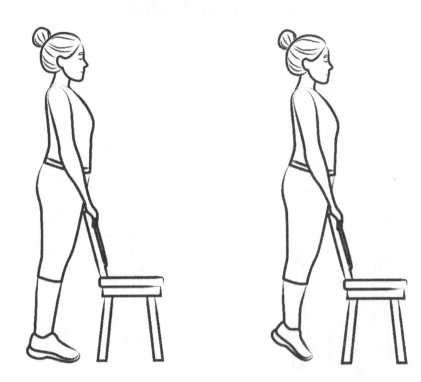

Purpose:

This exercise strengthens the calf muscles, improves ankle stability, and can help with balance.

Execution:

- Begin standing behind your chair, resting your hands on the backrest of the chair.
- Press down into the balls of both feet to raise your heels as high as you can.
- Hold for a moment at the top, then slowly lower your heels back to the floor.
- Repeat for a set of 10-15 repetitions.

CARDIO EXERCISES

42. SEATED MARCH

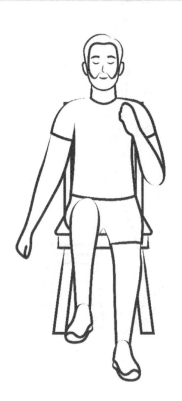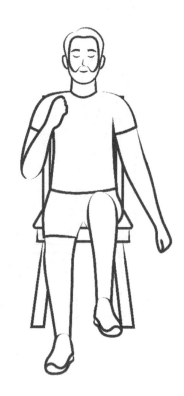

Purpose:

Seated March is a great way to boost circulation and strengthen leg muscles. It also offers a cardiovascular workout.

Execution:

- Begin by sitting comfortably on a chair with your spine straight, feet flat on the ground, and hands resting on your thighs or by your sides.
- As you lift your right knee towards your chest, swing your left arm forward in a controlled manner, similar to a marching motion.

- Gently lower your right foot back to the ground and bring your left arm back to its starting position. Now, as you lift your left knee towards your chest, swing your right arm forward.

- Gently lower your left foot back to the ground and return your right arm to its starting position.

- Alternate between the right and left legs, mimicking a marching motion while seated, and coordinating with the opposite arm.

- Continue this marching sequence for a set number of repetitions or for a specific duration, maintaining a steady rhythm.

43. SIDE LEG RAISES

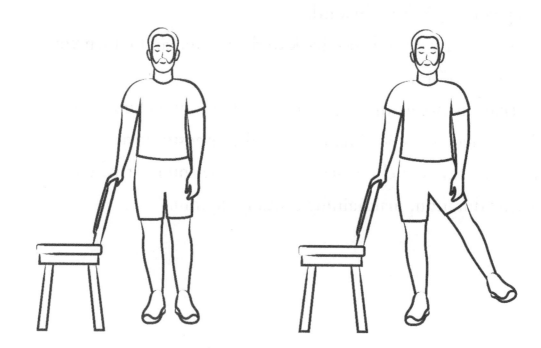

Purpose:

Develops strong hip and upper thigh muscles, which improve overall balance and stability.

Execution:

- Stand upright with a chair on your right, keeping your shoulders relaxed and arms resting on your sides.
- Place your left hand on your waist and grab the chair with your right hand for support and balance.
- Lift your left leg out to the side by engaging your core and thigh muscles, keeping it straight.
- Hold this position for a few seconds before slowly lowering your leg back down.
- Repeat the movement for 5 repetitions before switching sides and repeating the movement with the right leg.

44.   SEATED JUMPING JACKS

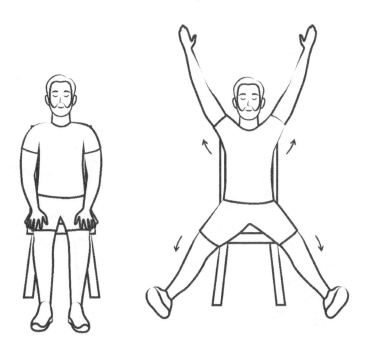

Purpose:

Increases heart rate and breathing, which improves cardiovascular health.

Execution:

- Sit on your chair and engage your core by drawing your belly button toward your spine.
- Take a deep breath in and extend your legs out to the sides, simultaneously lifting your arms up and out to the sides.
- Your legs and arms should form a "V" shape.
- Exhale and return to the starting position by bringing your legs and arms back. Repeat for 5 to 10 repetitions, maintaining a controlled and fluid motion.
- Throughout the exercise, keep your core engaged, posture upright, and avoid slouching or leaning back into the chair.
- Gradually increase the range of motion and intensity of the movement as you become more comfortable and proficient with the exercise.

45. BICYCLE CRUNCHES

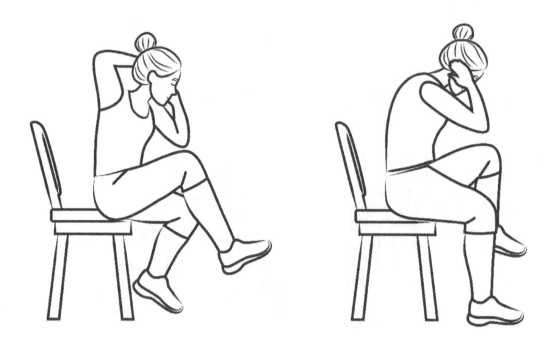

Purpose:

Strengthens the core muscles, especially the oblique muscles, which support fat burning and weight loss.

Execution:

- Lift your right knee towards your chest while simultaneously bringing your left elbow towards it as you crunch and slightly twist your body by engaging your core muscles.

- Try to go as close as possible to touching your right knee to your left elbow and hold this position for a moment.

- Then, lower your knee back to the floor and lift your torso back up to sit straight.

- Wait for a breath and repeat on the other side (left knee to right elbow).

- Aim to alternate between the two sides for 5-10 repetitions, slowly increasing the range of your motion and speed of the movement as you get used to it.

46. MODIFIED MOUNTAIN CLIMBERS

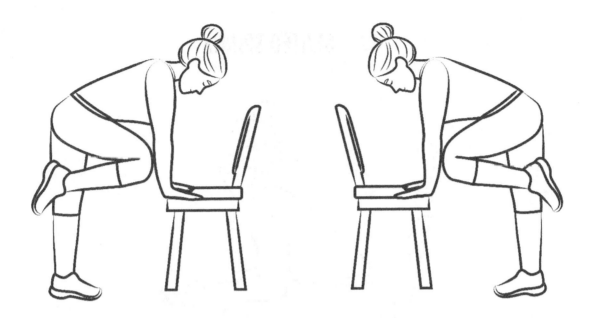

Purpose:

Strengthens core and leg muscles, increases heart rate that helps to burn calories, and aids in weight loss.

Execution:

- Stand in front of a chair with your feet shoulder distance apart.
- Gently bend forward at your hips to lower your torso closer to the chair and place the palms of your hands on the seat of the chair.
- Next, take a deep inhale and bring your right knee close to your arms. If you can manage to touch your elbows, that's great, but do not worry if you can't, and just focus on improving your range of motion over time.
- Lower your right foot back to the ground and repeat with the other leg.
- Aim for 5 to 10 continuous alternating repetitions for 3 sets.

MEDITATION EXERCISES

47. SEATED SPHINX

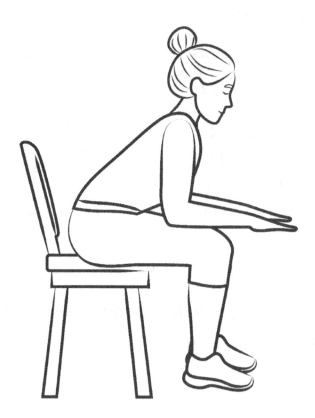

Purpose:

Opens up the chest, which supports respiratory function by allowing the lungs to expand fully.

Execution:

- Bend forward at the hips while keeping your back straight as you slide your hands forward on your thighs.
- Simultaneously, lower your elbows to place them on your thighs. Continue bending forward until your elbows are directly below your shoulders and you form a 90-degree bend in your arms.

-   Lift your chest slightly to form a slight curve in your back. Remember to keep your neck elongated and your head aligned with your spine.

-   Avoid any strain or tension in your neck by keeping it relaxed. Hold the pose for 5 breaths, inhaling and exhaling steadily. Allow your breath to flow naturally and maintain a sense of relaxation throughout the pose.

-   Release the pose by lifting your torso back into the starting position and then repeat for up to 3 repetitions, focusing on maintaining smooth movement.

48.   LOTUS POSE

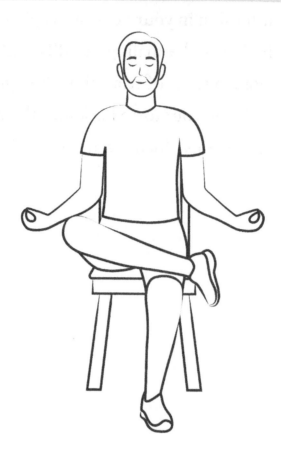

Purpose:

Classic "calm down" yoga pose with a slight chair modification.

Execution:

- Sit on a chair with your feet on the floor and your spine straight. Relax your shoulders and place your hands on your knees.
- Lift your right foot and place it on top of your left knee.
- Flex your right knee and gently press it down towards the ground, maintaining a straight spine and relaxed shoulders.
- Rest your hands on your knees, palms facing up or down.
- Take a few deep breaths and allow your body to relax in this position.
- Switch your legs halfway through the practice to balance out the stretch.

49. SUN BREATHS

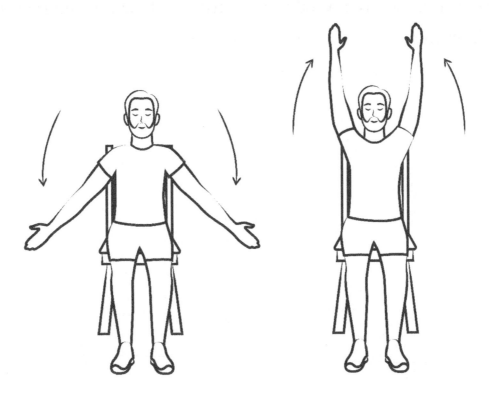

Purpose:

The Sun Breaths pose offers a serene way to anchor oneself while deepening the connection to one's breathing.

Execution:

- Start by positioning yourself upright on a chair, ensuring your feet are firmly planted on the floor and spaced hip-width apart.
- Maintain a straight spine and let your shoulders ease into a relaxed stance.
- Initiate the exercise by drawing a deep breath in through your nostrils, allowing the inhalation to guide your movements.
- As you breathe in, lift your arms in a sweeping motion with palms facing forward. Ensure your shoulders remain at ease as you extend your arms overhead.
- When exhaling, release the breath through your nostrils slightly before you begin to lower your arms.

- Slightly rotate your palms outward as you gracefully bring your arms back down to your sides.
- Continue this pattern several times, letting each breath and movement bring you closer to a state of calm and centeredness.

50. PRAYER POSE

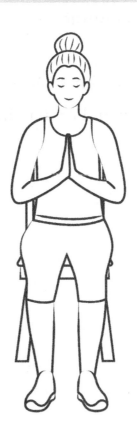

Purpose:

Beyond fostering breath mindfulness, this pose provides a gentle stretch to the upper torso, encouraging improved posture.

Execution:

- Start by positioning yourself upright on a chair, ensuring your feet are firmly planted on the floor and spaced hip-width apart.
- Maintain a straight spine and let your shoulders ease into a relaxed stance.
- Initiate the exercise by drawing a deep breath in through your nostrils, allowing the inhalation to guide your movements.
- As you breathe in, lift your arms in a sweeping motion with palms facing forward. Ensure your shoulders remain at ease as you extend your arms overhead.

- When exhaling, release the breath through your nostrils slightly before you begin to lower your arms.

- Slightly rotate your palms outward as you gracefully bring your arms back down to your sides.

- Continue this pattern several times, letting each breath and movement bring you closer to a state of calm and centeredness.

51. THE GODDESS POSE

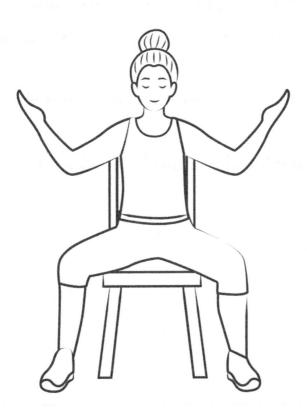

Purpose:

A grounding pose that focuses on opening the chest and shoulders while also increasing the hip's range by stretching the adductors.

Execution:

- Spread your hips as wide as possible while splaying your feet.
- Make sure your knees are directly above your feet for proper alignment. If you have reached your maximum hip range and your knees are collapsing inward, slightly narrow your stance to correct.
- Once you are in position, move your legs outward until you feel a strong but controlled stretch. Now that your legs are in position, raise both arms laterally (out to your sides) until they are just below shoulder height, with your palms facing up.

- Bend both your arms at the elbows until they are at 90 degrees or less. Now that your arms are in position, draw your shoulder blades back and downward while lifting your chest and lengthening your neck.

- Once in the position, you will feel your chest opening outward and your spine extending.

- Now you are in a full Goddess pose, draw your abs inward to fully engage your core muscles.

- Close your eyes and breathe normally for 15 to 20 breaths before releasing.

52. CHAKRA

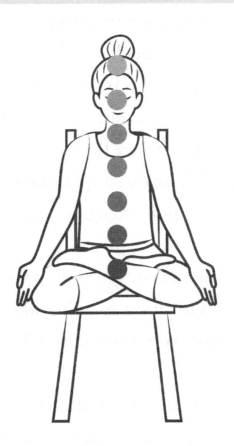

Purpose:

Advanced meditation technique to deepen your practice and enhance spiritual growth.

Chakras are energy centers in the body, and seven main ones are located from the base of the spine to the top of the head, representing a different aspect of our being.

Execution:

- Sit comfortably in a cross-legged position on a chair with your back straight, close your eyes, and take a few deep breaths, allowing yourself to relax.
- Begin by bringing your attention to the base of your spine, where the first chakra, the Root Chakra or Muladhara, is located. Visualize a spinning wheel

of vibrant red energy in this area, flowing freely and evenly, grounding you to the earth.

- Move your focus up to the lower abdomen, where the second chakra, Sacral Chakra or Svadhisthana, is located.

- Visualize a spinning wheel of orange energy, expanding and flowing harmoniously, enhancing your creativity and passion.

- Next to the upper abdomen, where the third chakra, the Solar Plexus Chakra or Manipura, is situated. Visualize a spinning wheel of yellow energy in this area, empowering you and strengthening your personal power and confidence.

- Then to the center of your chest, where the fourth chakra, the Heart Chakra or Anahata, is located. Visualize a spinning wheel of vibrant green energy in this area, radiating love, compassion, and harmony, both inwardly and outwardly.

- Next, to the throat, where the fifth chakra, the Throat Chakra or Vishuddha, is situated. Visualize a spinning wheel of serene blue energy in this area, clearing your communication channels and allowing you to express yourself authentically.

- Move to the space between your eyebrows, where the sixth chakra, the Third Eye Chakra or Ajna, is located. Visualize a spinning wheel of deep indigo energy and connect it with your intuition and inner wisdom as this energy center expands.

- Finally, bring your attention to the top of your head, where the seventh chakra, known as the Crown Chakra or Sahasrara, is situated.

- Visualize a spinning wheel of brilliant violet or white energy in this area, connecting you to the divine. Allow the energy to flow freely through each chakra.

- If you notice any blockage or imbalance, visualize the energy becoming clear and harmonious in those areas.
- When you are ready to conclude the meditation, take a few deep breaths and gradually bring your awareness back to your physical body.
- Gently open your eyes and take a moment to reflect on your experience.

CHAPTER 5: 28 DAY CHALLENGE

Welcome to the 28-Day Challenge! There's no need to be intimidated – this challenge is flexible and can take you anywhere from 28 to 75 days. There's no shame in taking your time; remember, the only person you're racing is yourself.

The challenge is structured in three phases: the first 9 days are at a beginner level, days 10-21 are at an intermediate level, and days 22-28 are advanced exercises. This gradual progression ensures you build strength and confidence at your own pace.

"If you feel up to it, feel free to do an extra 1-2 rounds of the day's exercises or add morning/evening routine exercise throughout the day. The AM/PM exercises can be found on the following pages later in the book. On the other hand, if you feel like you haven't quite mastered the exercises, don't hesitate to repeat the first week for a second or even third time. There's no rush, and it's perfectly fine to take things slow"

Let's get started on this journey together!

Beginner Exercises

Day 1

Exercise	Number	Reps / Duration
Chair Cat-Cow Stretch	1	30s
Standing Wind Release	7	20s
Chair Child's Pose	8	20-30s
Seated twist	9	5 reps
Modified Push Up	35	10-20 reps
Seated March	42	10 reps
Seated Sphinx	47	free

Day 2

Exercise	Number	Reps / Duration
Neck Roll	2	30s
Seated forward bend	10	20-30s
Seated side stretch	11	5 reps
Chair lunge pose	12	20-30s
Leg Shuffle	36	10-20 reps
Side Leg Raises	43	5-10 reps
Lotus Pose	48	free

Day 3

Exercise	Number	Reps / Duration
Shoulder Shrugs	3	20s
Seated cactus pose	13	10 reps
Cobra pose	14	20-30s
Humble warrior pose	15	30s
Leg Raises	37	20 reps
Seated Jumping Jacks	44	5-10 reps
Sun Breaths	49	free

Day 4

Exercise	Number	Reps / Duration
Arm Circles	4	15 reps
Mountain Pose	16	20s
Standing Wind Release	7	20s
Chair Child's Pose	8	20-30s
Chair Squat	38	5-10 reps
Bicycle Crunches	45	10 reps
Prayer Pose	50	free

Day 5

Exercise	Number	Reps / Duration
Seated Urdhva Hastasana	5	5 reps
Seated twist	9	5 reps
Seated forward bend	10	20-30s
Seated side stretch	11	5 reps
Chair Dips	39	5 reps
Modified Mountain Climbers	46	10 reps
The Goddess Pose	51	free

Day 6

Exercise	Number	Reps / Duration
Leg Pendulums	6	10 reps
Chair lunge pose	12	20-30s
Seated cactus pose	13	10 reps
Humble warrior pose	15	30s
Shoulder Press	40	10-20 reps
Seated March	42	10 reps
Chakra	52	free

Day 7: Rest Day

Congratulations on completing your first week! Take a moment to reflect on how you feel and how the exercises have been for you. If you feel like you haven't quite gotten the hang of it yet, feel free to repeat the first week before moving forward with the challenge. On the other hand, if you feel up for more, go ahead and add an extra 1-2 rounds to your routine.

Keep listening to your body and enjoy the journey!

Day 8

Exercise	Number	Reps / Duration
Chair Cat-Cow Stretch	1	30s
Mountain Pose	16	20s
Standing Wind Release	7	20s
Chair Child's Pose	8	20-30s
Chair Supported Calf Raises	41	10-20 reps
Side Leg Raises	43	5-10 reps
Seated Sphinx	47	free

Day 9

Exercise	Number	Reps / Duration
Neck Roll	2	30s
Seated twist	9	5 reps
Seated forward bend	10	20-30s
Chair lunge pose	12	20-30s
Modified Push Up	35	10-20 reps
Seated Jumping Jacks	44	5-10 reps
Lotus Pose	48	free

Intermediate Exercises

Day 10

Exercise	Number	Reps / Duration
Shoulder Shrugs	3	20s
Standing Tree	17	10-20s
Standing Hastasan	18	3-5 reps
Praying Spinal Twist	19	5 reps
Leg Shuffle	36	10-20 reps
Bicycle Crunches	45	5-10 reps
Sun Breaths	49	free

Day 11

Exercise	Number	Reps / Duration
Arm Circles	4	15 reps
Chair Pigeon Pose	20	30s
Dancer Pose	21	30s
Chair Eagle Pose	22	30s
Leg Raises	37	20 reps
Modified Mountain Climbers	46	5-10 reps
Prayer Pose	50	free

Day 12

Exercise	Number	Reps / Duration
Seated Urdhva Hastasana	5	5 reps
Humble King Arthur's Pose	23	30s
Chair Warrior Pose	24	30s
Upward Plank	25	10-20s
Chair Squat	38	5-10 reps
Seated March	42	10 reps
The Goddess Pose	51	free

Day 13

Exercise	Number	Reps / Duration
Leg Pendulums	6	10 reps
Standing Tree	17	
Standing Hastasan	18	
Praying Spinal Twist	19	
Chair Dips	39	5 reps
Side Leg Raises	43	5-10 reps
Chakra	52	free

Day 14: Rest Day

Congratulations on reaching the end of your second week! Reflect on your progress and how you're feeling. If you feel like you need more time with the intermediate exercises, don't hesitate to repeat the second week before moving on. If you're feeling strong and capable, consider adding an extra 1-2 rounds to your routine. Keep pushing yourself, but always listen to your body.

Day 15

Exercise	Number	Reps / Duration
Chair Cat-Cow Stretch	1	30s
Chair Pigeon Pose	20	30s
Dancer Pose	21	30s
Chair Eagle Pose	22	30s
Shoulder Press	40	10-20 reps
Seated Jumping Jacks	44	5-10 reps
Seated Sphinx	47	free

Day 16

Exercise	Number	Reps / Duration
Neck Roll	2	30s
Humble King Arthur's Pose	23	30s
Chair Warrior Pose	24	30s
Upward Plank	25	10-20s
Chair Supported Calf Raises	41	10-20 reps
Bicycle Crunches	45	5-10 reps
Lotus Pose	48	free

Day 17

Exercise	Number	Reps / Duration
Shoulder Shrugs	3	20s
Standing Tree	17	10-20s
Standing Hastasan	18	3-5 reps
Praying Spinal Twist	19	5 reps
Modified Push Up	35	10-20 reps
Modified Mountain Climbers	46	10 reps
Sun Breaths	49	free

Day 18

Exercise	Number	Reps / Duration
Arm Circles	4	15 reps
Chair Pigeon Pose	20	30s
Dancer Pose	21	30s
Chair Eagle Pose	22	30s
Leg Shuffle	36	10-20 reps
Seated March	42	20-30s
Prayer Pose	50	free

Day 19

Exercise	Number	Reps / Duration
Seated Urdhva Hastasana	5	5 reps
Humble King Arthur's Pose	23	30s
Chair Warrior Pose	24	30s
Upward Plank	25	10-20s
Leg Raises	37	20 reps
Side Leg Raises	43	5-10 reps
The Goddess Pose	51	free

Day 20

Exercise	Number	Reps / Duration
Leg Pendulums	6	10 reps
Standing Tree	17	10-20s
Standing Hastasan	18	3-5 reps
Praying Spinal Twist	19	5 reps
Chair Squat	38	5-10 reps
Seated Jumping Jacks	44	5-10 reps
Chakra	52	free

Day 21: Rest Day

Great job completing three weeks of the challenge! Take some time to assess how you feel and how well you've adapted to the intermediate exercises. If you feel you need more practice with these exercises, feel free to repeat the second and third weeks. If you're feeling confident and ready for more, you can move on to the advanced exercises or add an extra 1-2 rounds to your sessions. Keep up the great work and stay motivated!

Advanced Exercises

Day 22

Exercise	Number	Reps / Duration
Chair Cat-Cow Stretch	1	30s
Low Lunge Pose	26	15-30s
Seated Cow Face	27	20s
Bridge Pose	28	20-30s
Chair Dips	39	5 reps
Bicycle Crunches	45	5-10 reps
Seated Sphinx	47	free

Day 23

Exercise	Number	Reps / Duration
Neck Roll	2	30s
Chair Plank	29	10-20s
Downward Dog Pose	30	20s
Pigeon Pose	31	20-30s
Shoulder Press	40	10-20 reps
Modified Mountain Climbers	46	10 reps
Lotus Pose	48	free

Day 24

Exercise	Number	Reps / Duration
Shoulder Shrugs	3	20s
Seated Side Lunge	32	30s
Triangle Pose	33	20s
Puppy Dog Pose	34	30s
Chair Supported Calf Raises	41	10-20 reps
Seated March	42	20-30s
Sun Breaths	49	free

Day 25

Exercise	Number	Reps / Duration
Arm Circles	4	15 reps
Low Lunge Pose	26	15-30s
Seated Cow Face	27	20s
Bridge Pose	28	20-30s
Modified Push Up	35	10-20 reps
Side Leg Raises	43	5-10 reps
Prayer Pose	50	free

Day 26

Exercise	Number	Reps / Duration
Seated Urdhva Hastasana	5	5 reps
Chair Plank	29	10-20s
Downward Dog Pose	30	20s
Pigeon Pose	31	20-30s
Leg Shuffle	36	10-20 reps
Seated Jumping Jacks	44	10 reps
The Goddess Pose	51	free

Day 27

Exercise	Number	Reps / Duration
Leg Pendulums	6	10 reps
Seated Side Lunge	32	30s
Triangle Pose	33	20s
Puppy Dog Pose	34	30s
Leg Raises	37	20 reps
Bicycle Crunches	45	10 reps
Chakra	52	free

Day 28 Rest Day

Congratulations on completing the 28-day Chair Yoga Challenge!

See the next page of the book for a surprise for you!

EXTRA BONUS

Congratulations on completing the 28-day Chair Yoga Challenge!

Now that you're a Chair Yoga master, you can personalize your routine even further.

Feel free to **add extra rounds** to the advanced exercises, **combine** them with your morning or evening routines (which are on the following pages later in the book), or try **incorporating** some exercises from your extra bonus.

As a reward for your dedication and hard work, I would like to give you a FREE **"WALL PILATES WORKOUTS"** book.

You heard that right. Whole new book. For FREE!

To claim your free book, simply scan the QR code below or enter this link into your browser:

https://bit.ly/WP-Free-Bonus

Morning Chair Yoga Routine 1

Welcome to your morning Chair Yoga routine! This sequence is designed to be the perfect start to your day, consisting of activation exercises that will wake up your body and prepare you for the day ahead.

You should perform this routine in 3 sets, holding each exercise for approximately 20 seconds. This structure ensures you get the most benefit from each movement, helping you feel energized and ready to take on the day.

AM ROUTINE

1. CHAIR CAT-COW STRETCH

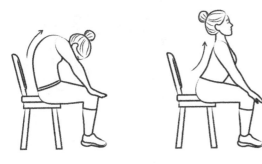

9. SEATED TWIST

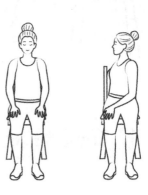

11. SEATED SIDE STRETCH

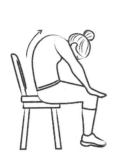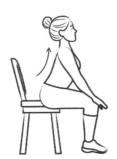

Morning Chair Yoga Routine 2

You should perform this routine in 3 sets, holding each exercise for approximately 20 seconds. This structure ensures you get the most benefit from each movement, helping you feel energized and ready to take on the day.

AM ROUTINE

10. SEATED FORWARD BEND

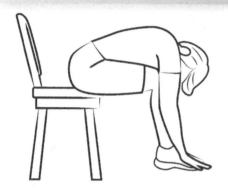

14. COBRA POSE

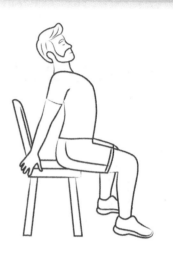

17. STANDING TREE

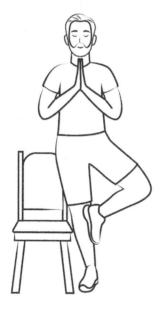

Morning Chair Yoga Routine 3

You should perform this routine in 3 sets, holding each exercise for approximately 20 seconds. This structure ensures you get the most benefit from each movement, helping you feel energized and ready to take on the day.

AM ROUTINE

49. SUN BREATHS

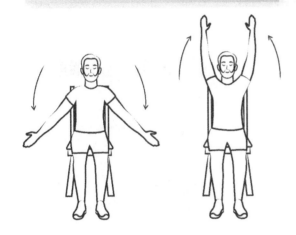

13. SEATED CACTUS POSE

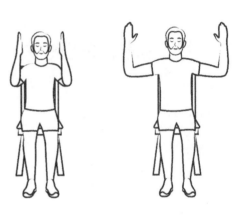

21. DANCER POSE

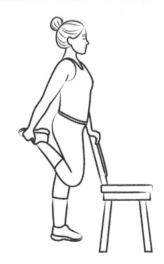

Evening Chair Yoga Routine 1

Welcome to your evening Chair Yoga routine! This sequence is centered around meditative exercises that will help you unwind and relax after a long day, preparing your mind and body for a restful night's sleep.

You should perform this routine in 3 sets, holding each exercise for approximately 20 seconds. This structure ensures you get the most benefit from each movement, helping you to calm your mind and soothe your body before bedtime.

PM ROUTINE

22. CHAIR EAGLE POSE

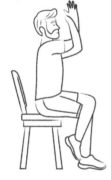

47. SEATED SPHINX

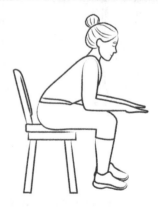

50. PRAYER POSE

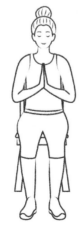

Evening Chair Yoga Routine 2

You should perform this routine in 3 sets, holding each exercise for approximately 20 seconds. This structure ensures you get the most benefit from each movement, helping you to calm your mind and soothe your body before bedtime.

PM ROUTINE

8. CHAIR CHILD'S POSE

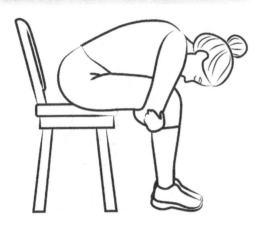

51. THE GODDESS POSE

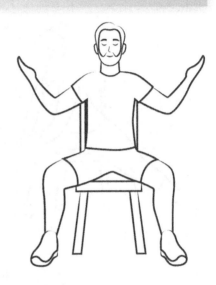

47. SEATED SPHINX

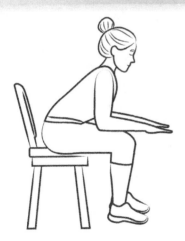

Evening Chair Yoga Routine 3

You should perform this routine in 3 sets, holding each exercise for approximately 20 seconds. This structure ensures you get the most benefit from each movement, helping you to calm your mind and soothe your body before bedtime.

PM ROUTINE

15. HUMBLE WARRIOR POSE

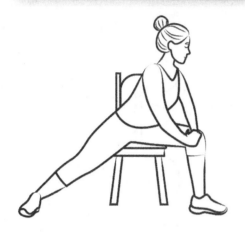

48. LOTUS POSE

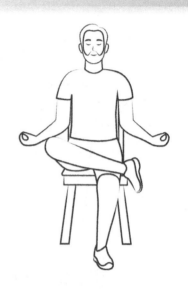

5. SEATED URDHVA

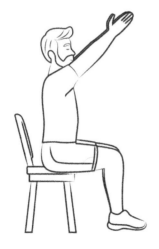

BONUS CHAPTER 1: MEDITATION

In meditation, the mind is clear, relaxed, and inwardly focused. When you meditate, you are fully awake and alert, but your mind is not focused on the external world or on the events taking place around you.

—Lama Surya Das

The power of the mind over the body is a force to be reckoned with, and meditation allows you to tap into that power. Meditative practices have a resounding impact on the way your inner self manifests. Finding that sense of peace within yourself enables you to explore the deeper pits within your shadow self that you try to keep buried, and in doing so, you become a stronger and more resilient version of yourself.

Cultivating awareness of the self is imperative to reap the benefits of yoga, and meditation and yoga go hand in hand to allow you to reach that degree of self-awareness. Knowing the elements that define you can help you work on your growth and become a superior version of your former self.

Augmenting the Mind–Body Connection

Yoga and meditation have a considerable overlap in cultivating a sense of inner peace. While yoga focuses on physical movements and dedication to the postures (asana), meditation focuses on the mental realm. Meditation helps you clear your mind of everyday clutter. It helps to sow the seeds of inner peace and the ability to find yourself and conquer it. When you conquer your weaknesses and everything that holds you back from becoming the person you want to be, the path ahead of you illuminates and leads you to your destination. You become more satisfied with yourself, and the goals you once set for yourself become more tangible.

A sense of inner stillness is necessary to concentrate on any task. This is why the significance of meditation cannot be weighed lightly on any scale. If you meditate daily, your focus improves and the turnaround time of any task allocated to you is shortened.

It is preferable to meditate before you perform yoga. This is because it clears up your mind and helps you focus more intently on the postures of yoga, also known as asanas. Moreover, it can help you feel energetic. Mindfulness is a highly sought-after attribute for your personality and can be enhanced through meditation and yoga. Practicing both together daily produces a synergistic effect on an unimaginable scale. The connection between your mind and body grows and you find deeper contentment in your daily activities.

Together, meditation and yoga can help reduce stress significantly. Meditation calms the nerve centers and helps lower cortisol levels in the bloodstream, which helps you feel more at peace with yourself. When you find a sense of inner peace, you tend to focus more easily on whatever you have to do and find joy in everything life has to offer. Additionally, you develop a positive outlook that helps you find an upside to every facet of life, even the calamities that befall you.

Emotional regulation is another byproduct of meditation. As a result of committing to a life composed of meditation, you tend to process the gamut of emotional situations in a way that contributes to your emotional intelligence. Expressing the right emotions in the face of life-changing events makes your social image more robust. Furthermore, it allows you to be aware of your hidden emotions that might interfere with daily activities. Acknowledging these emotions and regulating them becomes possible through meditation as you tap into the latent potential of your inner self. The power of your inner self is very potent, and meditation helps make it even more so to help you become strong enough to tackle anything life throws at you. This is why meditation is highly recommended for those of us who ardently commit to yoga practices.

How to Start

Find a quiet place and set a time limit for yourself. Sit cross-legged on the floor and focus on your body and breath. If your mind wanders, bring your attention back to your breath. If your mind wanders recursively, do not judge yourself, just return your focus to your breaths. Finally, open your eyes and listen to your surroundings. Notice how your body feels after this phase.

Try to commit to this practice at the same time every day and do it consistently. Moreover, work on increasing the time you spend meditating. If you start by meditating for 15 minutes every day, try increasing this time by 5 minutes every week.

BONUS CHAPTER 2: SLEEP

Yoga is the perfect opportunity to be curious about who you are. Sleep allows the inner exploration to deepen, rejuvenating the body and mind.

—Jason Crandell

Recent scientific discoveries have revealed the importance of sleep. Scientists argue that the body undergoes repair when asleep, allowing the cells to dispose of worn-out protoplasmic structures and make new ones. The brain processes and stores valuable experiences and important information learned throughout the day. More profound sleep leads to better lives wherein you enjoy every moment.

The Circadian Rhythm and Sleep Pattern

The circadian rhythm (biological clock) of your body makes you fall asleep at specific times, and you need to adhere to it to allow yourself some good sleep. Go to bed early and get up early in the morning to fully reap the benefits of yoga, as you cannot do so if your body is tired. You need to adjust your sleep pattern in a way that aligns with your natural circadian rhythm, which is the same for all of us and is about getting up to seven to eight hours of sleep a day. Try to go to bed and get up at the same time every day to regulate your biological clock.

Exposure to the Sun

Expose yourself to the sun as soon as you wake up so that the hormone serotonin surges through your bloodstream. Serotonin helps you feel energetic and full of vigor, which allows you to commit to your daily activities with greater energy. Serotonin levels in the body are subject to the regulation of the circadian rhythm.

If you have a massive disruption in your sleep pattern, you are likely to have your serotonin levels undergo fluctuations. This predisposes you to mood swings and results in a lack of energy to commit to everyday tasks, which is why adjusting your sleep routine is important.

Caffeine Intake

Caffeine intake can cause a serious disruption in the regulation of sleep patterns. Avoid consuming caffeine close to your bedtime or in the evenings. If you really need to drink coffee or tea, do it early in the day. Consuming any caffeinated drinks later in the day makes you subject to sleep disturbances. Some people might not be able to sleep at all after consuming coffee in the evening.

Shutting Out Sources of Disruption

Your bedroom is supposed to be a place where you can sleep without any disturbances. Therefore, it is better not to have a television or other sources of entertainment in this space. It is good if you happen to be someone who can exercise self-control, but many people cannot do this and succumb to the idea of watching a bit of their favorite program just when the clock ticks toward the time of hitting the hay. This habit can wreak havoc on your bedtime routine. Also, instead of watching TV, try to commit to a habit of bedtime rituals that predispose you to a more profound state of sleep. This can include having a warm bath before you go to bed. Warm showers calm the nerves and make you fall asleep.

The Importance of Bedtime Rituals

Disconnect from the internet and any devices around you. We do not realize the detrimental impact of social media and the internet on our sense of tranquility and productivity. Try disconnecting yourself from the web before you go to bed. Also, you can use some essential oils in your bedroom to help you fall asleep. Lavender oil can calm the nerves and help induce sleep. Commit to these habits to maximize the benefits of yoga. It is a good habit to get into reading books and novels before going to bed.

Ventilation in Your Bedroom

The flow of air into and out of your room has monumental importance. If hot air builds up in your space, especially during the summer season, you will eventually resort to using air conditioning more often, but you can cut down on that if you find time to let air pass through your room every day. This helps to cool down your room and prevent odors from developing due to inadequate ventilation.

Snacking at Bedtime

Always try to have your meals two or three hours before bed. Going to bed with a belly filled with food yet to be digested can lead to discomfort and reduced sleep quality.

The Integrity of Your Sleep Temple

Consider your bedroom your sleep temple. You'll need to remove television sets and any digital devices that keep you hooked to the internet. Also, when using screens, try to put on blue light filtering glasses, as blue light from screens can be a source of agitation. It is best to put your cellphone into airplane mode, so you are not disturbed by the EMF radiation during the night.

Spending Time in Nature

Devote some time to interact with nature, as this helps to regulate your biochemical processes. Go to the beach or spend time in a garden. This can really help soothe your senses and nerves. Even grounding yourself by walking barefoot can help you feel better. In fact, when your connection to the Earth is restored through grounding, electrons flood throughout your body, reducing inflammation and oxidative stress while also reinforcing your body's defense mechanisms. Electron transfers are the basis of virtually all antioxidant and anti-inflammatory activity. This is why spending time in nature can feel truly meditative and relaxing.

3 SECRET BONUSES

To get your ALL 3 SECRET BONUSES FOR FREE, just **scan the QR code above or enter this link**: https://bit.ly/3-secret-bonuses into your search browser.

Curious about the amazing gifts in your 3 BONUSES?

✓ Printable Yoga Chart with All the Exercises

✓ How to Create a Habit

✓ Simple Biohacks to Live Longer

And as a token of my appreciation, I'm also gifting you all my future books for free because I genuinely care about your journey.

Prepare to take your fitness to the next level!

Yours truly, Alex.

CONCLUSION

Committing to a yoga routine without any preparation might be akin to setting sail on a perilous voyage without having any proactive strategies on deck. Most people these days have developed a knack for health-related strategies that optimize their daily living. Turning your inclination for a healthy lifestyle into workable solutions requires dedication, and above all, a basic know-how of what you need to do to integrate these solutions into your life. Yoga is one such activity that requires utmost dedication to fulfill the goals that you set for yourself.

Thank you for allowing me to be part of your fitness journey. Remember, the only limit to your impact is your imagination and commitment. Keep moving forward!

I would greatly appreciate it if you could take a moment to leave a review. Your feedback not only helps me improve but also assists other readers in finding the guidance they need. Thank you for your support!

Alex

HELP ME SPREAD THE WORD

I hope you have been able to extract all the wisdom and knowledge from this book and put the challenges into action. Please don't forget to leave a review on Amazon, and let me know how this book has helped you. I would love to hear the transformation results that you have achieved after putting the content of this book into practice.

As a new author your reviews will serve as inspiration for me to create better material and motivate me to keep coming up with highly informative books that will help you achieve your goals.

It has been a pleasure to be your guide on your fitness journey. Continue striving for better health; I am rooting for you!

Alex Harper

REFERENCES

Bilski, R. (2019, February 25). *Dirgha pranayama: An introduction to 3 part breathing*. Yogapedia.com. https://www.yogapedia.com/dirgha-pranayama-an-introduction-to-three-part-breath/2/11311

Nadi shodhan pranayama | How to do & benefits of nadi shodhan. (2023, June 18). Artofliving.org. https://www.artofliving.org/in-en/yoga/pranayama/nadi-shodhan-alternate-nostril-breathing

Williams, S. (2019, April 24). *What Is chair yoga? Benefits, poses & more*. Yoga Practice. https://yogapractice.com/yoga/what-is-chair-yoga/

Made in the USA
Middletown, DE
05 September 2024